Shahrul Rahman

Effect of Bean Extract (Phaseolus vulgaris L) to LDL and Ox-LDL and Relation of Ox-LDL on LOX-1 Gene Polymorphism 3'UTR

Shahrul Rahman

Effect of Bean Extract (Phaseolus vulgaris L) to LDL and Ox-LDL and Relation of Ox-LDL on LOX-1 Gene Polymorphism 3'UTR

LAP LAMBERT Academic Publishing

Impressum / Imprint

Bibliografische Information der Deutschen Nationalbibliothek: Die Deutsche Nationalbibliothek verzeichnet diese Publikation in der Deutschen Nationalbibliografie; detaillierte bibliografische Daten sind im Internet über http://dnb.d-nb.de abrufbar.

Alle in diesem Buch genannten Marken und Produktnamen unterliegen warenzeichen-, marken- oder patentrechtlichem Schutz bzw. sind Warenzeichen oder eingetragene Warenzeichen der jeweiligen Inhaber. Die Wiedergabe von Marken, Produktnamen, Gebrauchsnamen, Handelsnamen, Warenbezeichnungen u.s.w. in diesem Werk berechtigt auch ohne besondere Kennzeichnung nicht zu der Annahme, dass solche Namen im Sinne der Warenzeichen- und Markenschutzgesetzgebung als frei zu betrachten wären und daher von jedermann benutzt werden dürften.

Bibliographic information published by the Deutsche Nationalbibliothek: The Deutsche Nationalbibliothek lists this publication in the Deutsche Nationalbibliografie; detailed bibliographic data are available in the Internet at http://dnb.d-nb.de.

Any brand names and product names mentioned in this book are subject to trademark, brand or patent protection and are trademarks or registered trademarks of their respective holders. The use of brand names, product names, common names, trade names, product descriptions etc. even without a particular marking in this work is in no way to be construed to mean that such names may be regarded as unrestricted in respect of trademark and brand protection legislation and could thus be used by anyone.

Coverbild / Cover image: www.ingimage.com

Verlag / Publisher:
LAP LAMBERT Academic Publishing
ist ein Imprint der / is a trademark of
OmniScriptum GmbH & Co. KG
Heinrich-Böcking-Str. 6-8, 66121 Saarbrücken, Deutschland / Germany
Email: info@lap-publishing.com

Herstellung: siehe letzte Seite /
Printed at: see last page
ISBN: 978-3-659-67301-6

Zugl. / Approved by: Medan, University of Sumatera Utara, Dissertation, 2014

This book dedicated to my heaven's angel

Maiyuzalina and my beloved child

Ahmad Mujahid Anwar, Fatimah Zahra,

Nabila Humairah and Yusuf Shahrul Anwar

PREFACE

Finally my book with the title of Effect of Bean Extract (*Phaseolus vulgaris* L) to LDL and Ox-LDL and Relation of Ox-LDL on LOX-1 Gene Polymorphism 3'UTR188CT can be issued.

I would like to thank you and my gratitude to Allah for permission and health that given to me. Also thanks to my lovely wife and children for the encouragement at every turn. A big thank you also wants me give to rector UMSU, Agussani PhD, and dean of the medical faculty UMSU, Ade Taufiq MD, and staff on all the ease that has been given to me.

My thanks also to all teachers who has been guiding and providing knowledge and insight to add to my knowledge. Also my gratitude to LAMBERT Academic Publishing and specially Mr. Andrei Gisca as Acquisition Editor for his kind to review my book.

Hopefully this book can provide a valuable contribution to the development of science and useful for many people.

ABSTRACT

Background: Atherosclerosis is an inflammatory disease that leads to the emergence of aterom plaque, which causes thickening of the blood vessel wall. Acute myocardial infarction (AMI) is caused by rupture of atherosclerotic plaques that trigger acute thrombosis cause total occlusion of the coronary artery. Initiating event in atherosclerosis is the change LDL into oxidized (OxLDL). Activation of OxLDL would be mediated by various scavenger receptors, such as LOX-1. Consumption of legumes can reduce the risk of coronary heart disease. This study want to find out whether the kidney beans that are included in legumes have efficacious as preventive risk of atherosclerosis.

Objective: To prove that kidney bean extract can lower LDL and OxLDL plasma in LOX-1 gene polymorphism 3'UTR188C/T as preventive risk of atherosclerosis.

Research methods: laboratory experiments with phytochemical test, test kidney bean extract effect with a dose of 400 mg, 800 mg dan 1200 mg per day on lipid profile and plasma levels of OxLDL by Enzyme -linked Immunosorbent Assay (ELISA), test 3'UTR188C/T gene polymorphism with restriction enzyme.

Results: The results of the phytochemical screening kidney bean extract contain active compounds such as alkaloids, saponins, flavonoids, triterpenoids/steroids, and glycosides. LDL found decrease in all treatment groups with the highest decrease in the 800 mg group, although not significantly. But found elevated levels of OxLDL in all treatment groups with the highest increase were also in the group of 800 mg. Most study participants were genotype CT.

Conclusion: It has been produced kidney bean extract in the form of extracts condensed that has met the standards. Kidney bean extract can lower LDL cholesterol. Although kidney bean extract can increase plasma Ox-LDL, further research needs to be done to see the existence of an increase in the levels of OxLDL. Participants with TT genotype had higher levels of plasma OxLDL than other genotypes.

Keywords :   Kidney bean extract, LDL level, Ox-LDL level, genotype, atherosclerosis

CONTENT

CHAPTER I
INTRODUCTION

1.1 Background

Atherothrombotic disease is the leading cause of death and morbidity of this disease is high. Although it may involve blood vessels all over the place in the body, but the main problem if induce clinical manifestations of coronary heart disease (CHD), cerebrovascular disease and peripheral arterial disease in the lower extremities.[1,2]

Atherosclerosis, a blockage of the arteries, is the result combination of abnormalities lipoprotein metabolism, oxidative stress, chronic inflammation and the possibility for the occurrence of thrombosis. This whole process will play a role in the onset of cardiovascular disease.[3-6]

Cardiovascular disease is the leading cause of death in most developed countries. Based on the results of basic health research in Indonesia on 2013, found the prevalence of CHD were diagnosed by a doctor or physician diagnosis or symptoms was 0.5% and 1.5%. CHD prevalence was higher in the community uneducated and not working. Most deaths from cardiovascular disease can be prevented through lifestyle changes such as diet, exercise, and stop smoking. For example, approximately 37% of heart attacks in women were associated with overweight. Moreover, hypercholesterolemia, which is a risk factor for cardiovascular disease can be overcome through proper diet in approximately 75% of individuals. Decrease input saturated fat; cholesterol and increased input of cholesterol-lowering foods such as nuts should be given priority as prevention for cardiovascular disease. Weight loss will also affect the increase in the production of superoxide dismutase (SOD) which would prevent LDL oxidation.[7-10]

Recent studies on atherosclerosis focus on inflammatory processes, thus providing a new picture mechanism of this disease. Inflammatory cytokines involved in the inflammatory process of the blood vessels to

1

stimulate the formation of endothelial adhesion molecules, proteases, and other mediators, which can enter the blood circulation in the dissolved form. These cytokines induce the production of interleukin-6, which will stimulate the liver to increase the production of acute phase reactants such as C-reactive protein. In addition, platelets and adipose tissue can induce inflammatory mediators, causing further atherothrombotic[11]

In recent decades, the understanding of the pathogenesis of atherosclerosis has been revolutionized. Previously estimated atherosclerosis has basic problems with the blood vessels alone. The understanding of the pathophysiology of this disease has entered a new era with the understanding pathobiology further atherothrombotic.[11]

Initial event in atherosclerosis is change low density lipoprotein (LDL) into a form that oxidized low density lipoprotein (Ox-LDL) by several factors such as radicals, lypooxygenation, causing fragmentation of unsaturated fatty acids into LDL particles. Oxidized LDL plays an important role in the development of atherosclerosis. Activity of oxidized LDL mediated by different receptors called scavenger receptor (SR), such as the SR-AI / II, SR-BI, CD36, MARCO, marcosialin (CD68) and lectin-like oxidized low-density lipoprotein receptor-1 (LOX- 1). Sawamura, et al, (1997), was first identified LOX-1 as the main receptor for endothelial cells in oxidized LDL[12-14]

Lectin-like oxidized low-density lipoprotein receptor-1 (LOX-1) has been known as a membrane protein with the ability to bind and degrade oxidized LDL. In vascular smooth muscle cells, oxidized LDL induces apoptosis through ROS generation. Apoptosis induced by oxidized LDL is also mediated by LOX-1 in human umbilical vein endothelial cells. Apoptosis or programmed cell death will create oxidative species that serves as inflammation that will contribute to atherosclerosis and cardiovascular disease.[14,15]

LOX-1 belongs to the subgroup of scavenger receptor class E, which is a human gene with a C-type lectin gene cluster on chromosome 12 containing genes receptor to recognize the immune system. Mango, et al, delivered until now there are 7 polymorphisms that have been identified in the LOX-1 gene. One is 3'UTR188C / T (T to C substitution at 3'untranslated region located at 188 bp). Chen, et al, found that the frequency of allele 3'UTR / T was significantly increased with an increase in the severity of stenosis in coronary artery disease in white women, while the black woman was not found significantly increased, which is likely influenced by the number of samples small. The same result was found by Mango, et al, that the polymorphism 3'UTR188C / T showed a significant association when compared between patients with acute myocardial infarction and normal controls. While Kurnaz, et al, found that the gene polymorphism 3'UTR188C / T as predisposing the development of left ventricular hypertrophy on coronary artery disease.[12,13,16,17]

Dry beans and soybeans are unique because that food rich in nutrients. The addition of nuts in the diet can lower blood cholesterol levels. Nuts contain complex carbohydrates, vegetable protein, dietary fibre, oligosaccharides, phytochemicals (especially isoflavones in soy), and minerals. Complex carbohydrates and fibre-containing foods contribute because it has a low glycemic index, which is beneficial for people with diabetes and reduce the risk for developing diabetes. The protein contained in soy is now recognized as a complete protein. Vegetables that used to replace animal protein may reduce urinary calcium excretion and reduce the risk for developing osteoporosis. Components of diets containing fibre, both soluble and insoluble, provide many health benefits. The importance of prebiotics as oligosaccharides and its role in the function of the colon have been widely recognized. Then, a mineral found in nuts is important to reduce the risk for osteoporosis and hypertension.[18,19]

Beans (Phaseolus vulgaris L) are a type of legume that has been known to have a diuretic effect and efficacy. Composition of beans are: folate, fibre, alkaloids, flavonoids, saponins, triterpenoida, steroid, stigmasterin, trigonelin, arginine, an aminoacid, asparagine, kholina, tannins, fasin, starch, vitaminA, vitamin C and minerals (copper, magnesium, iron, potassium, calcium).[20,21]

In addition, dry beans have also been shown to improve serum lipid profile in patients with coronary heart disease. The content of phytosterols from beans is approximately125 mg per 100 grams of beans.[22]

Based on the above description, throughout on the literature search conducted by researchers, research on the effects of bean extract that influence the inflammatory parameters, in this case the levels of LDL and oxidized LDL and its relation with LOX-1 gene polymorphisms 3'UTR188C / T, as a preventative measure risk of atherosclerosis has not been investigated. Therefore, this study will conduct phytochemical test to determine the class of the active compounds from the extract of beans; determine the frequency distribution of LOX-1 gene polymorphisms 3'UTR188C / T in Medan, examines the effects of bean extract on LDL and oxidized LDL levels and its relation with LOX-1 gene polymorphisms 3'UTR188C / T on the subject studied.

1.2 Problem formulation

Based on the background described previously, problem that will be the research questions are as follows:

1. Is the LOX-1 gene polymorphism 3'UTR188C / T is found in Medan?
2. Is there a relationship between the levels of LDL and oxidized LDL with LOX-1 gene polymorphism 3'UTR188C / T?
3. Does bean extract has an effect that can affect the levels of LDL and oxidized LDL and its relation with LOX-1 gene polymorphisms 3'UTR188C / T in humans?

1.3 Research objectives

1.3.1 General purpose

Role of bean extract in the prevention risk of developing atherosclerosis in normal subjects who differ in LOX-1 gene polymorphism 3'UTR188C / T.

1.3.2 Specific objectives

a. Determine the frequency distribution of LOX-1 gene polymorphisms 3'UTR188C / T in subjects studied

b. Determine the effect of bean extract and oxidized LDL cholesterol levels

c. Determine the relationship between changes in LDL and oxidized LDL levels by genotype subjects

1.4 Benefits research

1.4.1. Theoretical benefits: Result of this research is expected that beans can affect the levels of LDL and oxidized LDL on LOX-1 gene polymorphism 3'UTR188C/T in humans.

1.4.2. Benefits applicable:

a. Expected from the results of this study can help people to consume more beans because it has a good effect for protection against heart disease.

b. This study is a preliminary study, which is expected for universities to develop research on traditional materials as a nutritious plant pharmacological

1.5 Originality

Based on literature-based assessments in English as well as publications that have been abstracted in English, researchers have not found research on the effects of extracts of bean (Phaseolus vulgaris L.) against levels of LDL and oxidized LDL on LOX-1 gene polymorphism

5

3'UTR188C / T. Which have been studied are the effects of bean on the lipid profile and blood sugar levels.

1.6 The potential of intellectual property rights (IPR)

a. Getting the frequency distribution of LOX-1 gene polymorphisms 3'UTR188C / T on the subject in the field
b. Proving bean extract affects the levels of LDL and oxidized LDL in subjects carriers of LOX-1 gene polymorphisms 3'UTR188C / T.
c. The discovery of a new phytopharmaca formula that effective and safe in influencing levels of LDL and Ox-LDL

CHAPTER II
LITERATURE

2.1 Atherosclerosis

2.1.1 Definition

Atherosclerosis is a fibro proliferative complex inflammatory response on the retention of atherogenic lipoproteins in the arterial intima layer. Atherosclerosis is a chronic disease and a major cause of coronary heart disease and cardiovascular disease. On the origin of the word, atherosclerosis comes from the Greek, which is meaningful athere is porridge and skleros is hard.[2,23,24]

From that word, it can be concluded that atherosclerosis is the formation of spots like porridge consisting of fatty deposits of cholesterol in the intima layer of the blood vessel lumen. This situation resulted in the thickening of the walls blood vessels and loss of elasticity of the arteries, accompanied by changes in the media and intima layer degeneration.[2]

Atherosclerosis is a disease which is chronic inflammation of blood vessels, which causes the appearance of plaques atherom is a focal lesion located in the intima of blood vessels both large and medium. Retention of sub endothelial LDL and the oxidative cause beginning of atherogenesis, which is followed by inflammatory cell infiltration and activation of blood. Ox-LDL activates endothelial cells by inducing the expression of adhesion molecules that mediate turnover and adhesions blood leukocytes (monocytes and T cells). After adhesion to the endothelium, leukocytes migrate into the intima. Monocytes are then transformed into macrophages that enhance the scavenger receptor activation leading to increased fat accumulation and formation of soap cells. Activation of macrophages causing the release of pro inflammatory cytokines, reactive oxygen species (ROS), proteolytic enzymes involved in matrix degeneration and eventually cause unstable atherosclerotic plaque.[25-27]

7

Atherosclerosis is not same like arteriosclerosis. Arteriosclerosis has a broad meaning, covering all diseases that can lead to hardening of the arteries, such as atherosclerosis, stenosis after angioplasty, and peripheral vascular disease. As already known, the atherosclerotic lesion is a layer of fat (fatty streaks) has been found in the aorta during foetal development, especially in foetuses whose mothers had high cholesterol levels. This is what may underlie many cases of myocardial infarction occur in individuals without having ischemic symptoms beforehand. Therefore, long-term effort is needed to prevent this disease and the consequences of this disease are very dangerous.[2,11]

2.1.2 Pathogenesis

Understanding of the pathophysiology of atherosclerosis always comes cholesterol theory. Age, cholesterol, and LDL cholesterol concentration is an indication of the risk for the occurrence of cardiovascular disorders in the future. Some individuals are more convenient for atherosclerosis (e.g., men more often than women).[2,11]

Acute myocardial infarction (AMI) is caused by atherosclerotic plaque rupture triggering acute thrombosis resulting in total occlusion of the coronary artery. Ehara, et al., reported that the plasma levels of oxidized LDL in patients with AMI increased approximately 3.5 times compared with control subjects.[28]

LDL cholesterol is a major risk factor for atherosclerosis. However, controversy persists about how the mechanism of high concentrations of LDL can lead to atherosclerosis and its complications. Most likely, which is supported by the results of laboratory and clinical data, showed that LDL modified by oxidation or glycation trigger an inflammatory response in the walls of arteries, thus stimulating many biological processes that play a role in the early events of atherosclerosis, development, and it complications. At this time it is known that oxidized LDL is involved in atherosclerosis through cell

8

formation soap. However, inflammation that occurs in cells involved in atherosclerosis has a lot of risk factors associated with atherosclerosis, such as smoking, insulin resistance/diabetes mellitus, and hypertension.[11,29]

2.1.3 The beginning and development of atherosclerotic lesions

Chronic inflammation has an important role in early atherosclerosis and inflammatory processes can occur at any stage of the disease. Fat layer has no symptoms but can develop into a complex lesion. The fat layer increases the content of lipoproteins in the intima, which later merged with components and extracellular matrix such as proteoglycans. This causes lipoprotein stuck in the intima, the isolated plasma antioxidant, thus turning it into oxidized. This oxidation modifies LDL particles composed of a mixture of incomplete, because either lipids or proteins can undergo modifications. Substances such as the modified lipoprotein particles can cause a local inflammatory response.[11,23,24,30-32]

Further lesions can cause narrowing of the lumen and cause clinical symptoms. Smooth muscle cells have been found in human intima during early atherogenesis, under a layer of fat that is growing. Oxidized LDL has been found in atherosclerotic plaques but not present in the abnormal intima.[2]

2.1.4 Risk Factors

Atherosclerosis is the result of complex interactions between genes and environment. Chronic inflammation is believed to be pathogenic factors of atherosclerosis in humans. Factor gene itself may cause symptomatic atherosclerosis but very rarely. Mostly, the genetic background raises the individual response to atherogenic factor gene and blood vessel wall weakness against atherogenic stimuli but very obvious environmental factors affect the speed of progression of the disease (plaque development) and therefore determine when coronary heart disease occur.[2,26,33]

Both innate immune system and the adaptive nature have an important role at the beginning or trigger for the inflammatory processes associated with atherosclerosis. The immune system is triggered by the interaction between lipoproteins which has been modified by the scavenger receptor that can cause vascular inflammation.[34-36]

Risk factors for atherosclerosis are divided into:[2,37]a. Modified, such as: diabetes or impaired glucose tolerance; Dyslipidemia: increased total cholesterol, LDL cholesterol levels, decreased HDL cholesterol levels; smoking; and hypertension. b. Not modified, such as: longevity; gender; genetic disorders, such as familial hypercholesterolemia; have a close relative who has some complications of atherosclerosis (such as CHD or stroke).

Diabetes is a condition where the fasting blood glucose level $\geq$ 126 mg/dl. Risk for all forms of cardiovascular disease, including coronary heart disease is increased in type-1 and type-2 diabetes. Mortality in diabetics who have coronary heart disease is higher than the non-diabetic.[38]

From all the above risk factors, high levels of LDL cholesterol are a major cause of atherosclerosis.[2]

The role of LDL cholesterol in atherogenesis process is also supported by a genetic disorder that causes increased serum LDL cholesterol levels significantly although other risk factors for CHD was not found. Examples of genetic disorders are homozygous and heterozygous familial forms of hypercholesterolemia.[39]

Epidemiological data indicate a strong relationship between low HDL cholesterol levels with increased morbidity and mortality from coronary heart disease. High levels of HDL cholesterol reduce the risk of CHD. Epidemiological data found that 1% decrease in HDL cholesterol levels are associated with increased risk of CHD 2-3%. Low levels of HDL cholesterol are an independent risk factor for the occurrence of CHD.[39]

There are several factors that give the role to the occurrence of dyslipidemia, such as: obesity, smoking, less physical activity and type 2 diabetes mellitus.[39]

Smoking gives a big role on the risk for developing CHD and other forms of cardiovascular disease. The relationship between smoking and CHD risk is dose-dependent and is found in both men and women. Smoking cessation lowers the risk of developing CHD and decrease of that risk starting at the first month after quit smoking.[40]

Some studies get a strong relationship between high blood pressure with risk of CHD. This relationship was found in both men and women with young and old age. Decreased blood pressure in hypertensive patients lowers the risk of developing CHD. It is also common in the elderly with isolated systolic hypertension.[41]

CHD risk increases gradually with age in both men and women. This occurs because of age is a reflection of the progressive accumulation of atherosclerosis, which is associated with exposure continues over the atherogenic risk factors both known and unknown.[42]

Increased risk associated with age becomes more significant in men aged 45 years and over, and women after menopause. Men have a greater risk for developing CHD than women at any age. The reason for the differences is not yet fully understood. Reason can be explained is in male patients found an increase in LDL cholesterol and blood pressure and a decrease in HDL cholesterol.[42]

CHD tend to occur in families and family history of coronary heart disease is a risk factor for CHD. CHD risk reported to range from 2-12 times higher in the first generation compared with the general population. Some studies found that the risk occurs independently of other risk factors.[39]

Risk for atheroscleros is increased fourfold when encountered two risk factors. Dyslipidemia, hypertension, and smoking at the same time increase the risk for atherosclerosis up to seven times.[37]

11

As already described, the initial event in atherosclerosis is change LDL into oxidized LDL by several factors such as radical and lypooxygenation, causing fragmentation of unsaturated fatty acids into LDL particles. Oxidized LDL are pro inflammatory and pro atherogenic and associated with the onset, development, and destabilization of atherosclerotic lesions. Oxidized LDL increases the expression of pro inflammatory enzyme, causing the entry of monocytes into the vessel wall and made vascular endothelial cell dysfunction. Oxidized LDL change macrophages to foam cells which is the atherosclerotic plaque. Plaque rupture causes acute complications that scary in atherosclerosis. In many cases, the lesions are dangerous due to acute thrombosis of the coronary arteries do not cause critical narrowing of the arteries, making identification using standard angiography is not a priority. In fact, today it was found that the activation of the inflammatory process compared with the degree of stenosis is more often the cause of plaque rupture and thrombosis trigger causing tissue ischemia.[11,43]

The development of monoclonal antibodies that bind to specific epitopes oxidation has shown the development of sensitive and specific measurements to measure the levels of oxidized LDL in the circulation.[44-46]

2.1.5. The role of LDL cholesterol

Epidemiological studies have shown that serum total cholesterol levels associated with atherosclerosis risk. This relationship has been observed in many populations around the world. Because the serum LDL cholesterol levels associated with total cholesterol levels in the population, then the relationship between atherosclerosis with serum LDL cholesterol levels were increased equally. Risk for atherosclerosis increased with increasing concentrations of LDL cholesterol (Figure 1).[37,47]

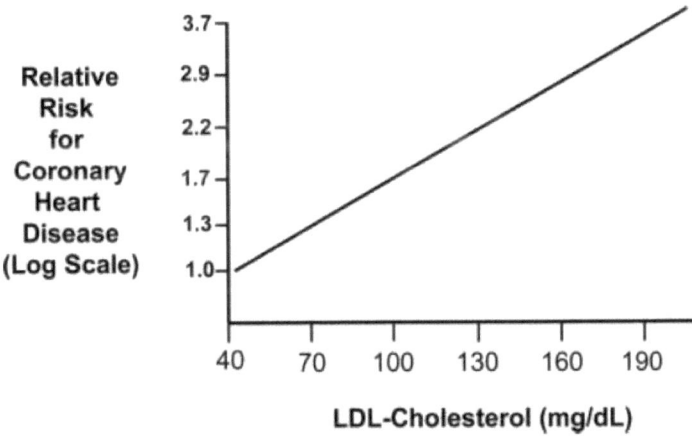

Figure1. Relationship straight line between LDL and the relative risk of coronary heart disease[37]

Figure 1 shows every change of 30 mg / dl LDL cholesterol, the relative risk for coronary heart disease changed approximately 30%.[37]

This relationship has two important implications: a. Those who have low LDL cholesterol levels that have the same absolute risk for the development of atherosclerosis with those who have high LDL cholesterol levels (due to other risk factors), it will have the same advantages if can decrease LDL cholesterol levels. b. Those that have low LDL cholesterol levels have lower absolute risk than those who have high LDL cholesterol levels have fewer benefits by lowering LDL cholesterol levels when their LDL cholesterol levels are low. [37]

The results of the Heart Protection Study (2002) also found strong evidence to support the relationship between LDL cholesterol levels and risk of coronary heart disease. Heart Protection Study concluded that the decrease in LDL cholesterol levels regardless of the initial value is lowers the risk in patients who have a high risk for atherosclerosis.[48]

2.1.6 LOX-1 as oxidized LDL receptor

Oxidized LDL works by binding to scavenger receptors such as SR-A, SR-BI, CD36, and lectin like oxidized low density lipoprotein receptor (LOX-1). LOX-1 has been identified as Ox-LDL receptor largest endothelial cells, although macrophages and smooth muscle cells also express LOX-1 in conjunction with other scavenger receptors.[49]

Oxidized LDL is believed to have an important role in the onset of atherosclerosis. One important factor that accelerates atherogenesis is the immune system that affects the process of atherosclerosis in the arterial wall. Oxidized LDL itself known by both the innate immune response and the adaptive. Oxidized LDL has several receptors such as SR-AI / II, SR-BI, CD 36, macrosialan, and CD 68. In 1997, the lectin-like oxidized LDL receptor-1 (LOX-1, OLR-1) has been identified from endothelial cells bovine aortic. LOX-1 is expressed and binds to oxidized LDL in peripheral tissues, including large artery endothelial cells, macrophages, and smooth muscle cells. Association of oxidized LDL to LOX-1 induces several cellular events in endothelial cells activation of transcription factors such as NF-κB, up regulation of monocyte chemoattractant protein-1 and reduction of intracellular nitric oxide, which triggers the occurrence of cardiovascular disorders or accelerate the development of atherosclerosis.[27,45,50-53]

Several studies have shown that oxidized LDL plays an important role in the pathogenesis of atherosclerosis. Oxidized LDL is also known to be immunogenic form a specific antibody that is anti-oxidized LDL. Not all oxidized LDL found in circulation as soon shifted by the reticuloendothelial system. Oxidized LDL that is in circulation will describe minimally modified LDL.[54-58]

Methods for evaluating the risk of developing atherosclerosis or to assess the status of the patient at this time already available. Among the methods that are invasive, Framingham score is most commonly used.

Another direct method is the measurement of carotid intima-media thickness and has been frequently used in observational studies. [59-61]

Oxidized LDL is involved in the early stages of atherogenesis, such as endothelial injury, the expression of adhesion molecules, and the retention and recruitment of leukocytes, as well as soap cell formation and thrombus. [62-63]

LOX-1 activation by oxidized LDL increases the levels of reactive oxygen species (ROS) through the action of NADPH oxidase. In vascular muscle cells, oxidized LDL induces apoptosis through ROS generation. ROS are molecules containing oxygen and has a higher reactivity than oxygen molecules, such as O2 and H2O2. ROS in low concentrations can activate signal transduction pathways and can alter expression of genes associated with growth and differentiation. Whereas at high concentrations, ROS have the effect to damage the cell. ROS are produced as a result of the body's normal metabolism in the mitochondria and the environment. When accompanied with less antioxidant abilities it can cause damage or oxidative stress. The result can be damage to deoxyribonucleic acid (DNA damage) which covers breakage or termination of the DNA chain, lipid peroxidation, protein modification, membrane disruption, and mitochondrial damage. ROS levels decreased in the presence of the antioxidant defence but increased by transition metal such as iron or copper, and by exogenous agents such as radiation and ozone. [64,65]

The reduced partial metabolism of oxygen molecules (O_2) is referred to as "reactive oxygen species" (ROS) caused by high reaction against O_2 molecules. ROS formed in intracellular through several processes, for example the results of normal aerobic metabolism and as second messengers in various signal transduction pathways. ROS can also be produced from exogenous extracellular material, or can also be produced as a result of exposure to certain environmental cell. [66,67]

Antioxidant defence mechanisms are not always adequately protect cells from ROS, if ROS exceeds the ability of cell antioxidants to prevent oxidative cell injury, then there cause of oxidative stress that can lead to various diseases in the human body. Oxidative stress can be defined as an increase in intracellular ROS exceeds the value ofphysiology.[68]

Oxidative stress stimulates the expression of protein kinases such as focal adhesion kinase and intercellular adhesion molecule (ICAM) - 1. Invasion of the arterial wall by monocytes and T lymphocytes are one of the early occurrences of atherosclerotic lesion development. Monocytes, macrophages, and smooth muscle cells have the scavenger receptor for oxidized LDL. Association of oxidized LDL causes activation of monocytes and macrophages and stimulates the expression of superoxide dismutase (SOD), which increases the concentration of hydrogen peroxide. This process is associated with excessive macrophage apoptosis and plays a role in the formation of atherosclerotic lesions. [66]

In endothelial cells, oxidized LDL-induced ROS production is dependent on the time and dose (dose and time dependent) and is mediated by LOX-1.Association of oxidized LDL to LOX-1 resulted in activation of NF-κB. Not working LOX-1 willnegate oxidized LDL-mediated activation of NF-κB on endothelial cells. ROS, which works as a second messenger, otherwise increase the expression of LOX-1. Oxidized LDL levels are also associated with small dense LDL and metabolic syndrome.[9,65,69,70]

Activation of NF-κB increase the migration and activation of neutrophils, platelets, lymphocytes, and NK cells to sites of inflammation through the production of Macrophage Colony Stimulating Factor (M-CSF), Granulocyte Colony Stimulating Factor (G-CSF), Granulocyte Macrophage Colony Stimulating Factor (GM- CSF), tissue factor, Vascular Cell Adhesion molecule-1 (VCAM-1), intercellular adhesion molecule-1 (ICAM-1), and *Endothelial Leucocytes Adhesion Molecule*-1 (ELAM-1). Besides, also produced pro inflammatory cytokines like TNF-α and the IL-1 that plays an important role in endothelial cell damage. Endothelial damage which occurs activate the process of thrombus formation in the lesion area, this leads to a narrowing of the vessel lumen. [68]

LOX-1 receptor is regulated by many factors that are part of the process atherosclerosis, including components of the immune system, cells located in the walls of arteries, oxidative substances, and intracellular processes. Figure 2 illustrates the complexity of the expression of LOX-1 pathway plays a role in the process of atherogenesis. [12,71]

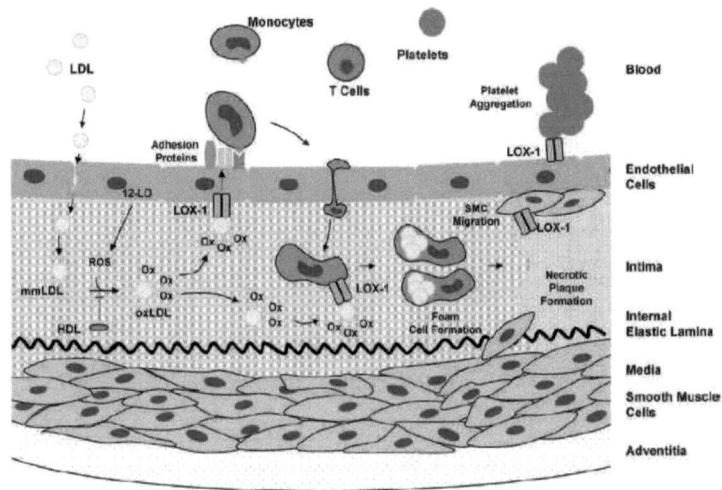

Figure 2. Participation of LOX-1 and oxidized LDL in atherosclerotic lesion formation. [12]

Figure 2 explained that the initial event in atherosclerosis is change LDL into oxidized LDL by several factors such as radical, lipooxygenation, causing fragmentation of unsaturated fatty acids into LDL particles. Oxidized LDL binding to the receptor LOX-1 stimulates the endothelial expression and secretion of enzymes such as MMPs pro atherogenic, in addition it also stimulated superoxide production. Increased MCP-1 and M-CSF will stimulates the development of plaque. This pro inflammatory state increases the expression of vascular adhesion molecules such as ICAM-1, P-selectin, E-selectin, PECAM-1 and VCAM-1. This led to the infiltration of monocytes

17

into the vessel wall. Monocytes that migrate into the blood vessels will differentiate into macrophages. These leukocytes also express scavenger receptors that mediate uptake of oxidized LDL. Macrophage lipid accumulation causes the formation of soap cells, causing cell death and the appearance of necrotic areas rich in fat. Cytokines can stimulate the proliferation and migration of smooth muscle cells to cover areas of necrosis forming fibrous lesions. Further modifications of these lesions cause calcification or plaque rupture and become involved in further atherothrombotic.[12,72]

Mango, et al., (2003), stated that there are currently seven polymorphisms that have been identified in the LOX-1 gene. The seventh polymorphisms are: Exon 4 K167N (501G> C), 3UTR 188C / T, Intron 4 IVS4 + 27 G> C. Intron 4 IVS4-73 C> T, Intron 4 IVS4-14 A> G, Intron 5 IVS5-70 A> G, Intron 5 IVS5-27 G>T.[16]

Kurnaz, et al., (2009), found that the K167N polymorphism is an independent risk factor of coronary artery disease compared with other cardiovascular risk factors.[73]Then in 2011, Kurnaz, et al., found that gene polymorphisms 3'UTR188C / T as predisposing of the development left ventricular hypertrophy on coronary artery disease.[11]

2.2Bean

Natural products are the main source of new drug development. Between the years 1981-2002, 5% of the 1,031 new drugs that have been approved by the USFDA is a natural product and 23% of other molecules contained in natural products.[74]

Simplicia medicinal plants are the raw materials for manufacturing extracts both as a medicinal ingredient or product. Simplicia is a natural substance that is used as a drug that has not undergone any treatment except in the form of dried material. Simplicia that used as raw materials must meet the requirements listed in the monograph published by the official

Ministry of Health (Materia Medical Indonesia) to produce standardized botanicals.

2.2.1 Taxonomy

Classification of bean plants according to the USDA 2008 is as follows: Kingdom : Plantae; Subkingdom : Tracheobionta; Division : Magnoliophyta; Class : Magnoliopsida; Subclass : Rosidae; Order : Fabales; Tribe: Fabaceae; Genus: Phaseolus; Species: Phaseolus vulgaris L

This plant is widely cultivated throughout the world include various forms of cultivation. Taxonomic division is usually based farming groups not based on botanical aspects. Here are 12 species of Phaseolus: a. Phaseolus acutifolius A. Gray - tepary bean: growing up in the Southwest US and Mexico. b. Phaseolus angustissimus A. Gray - slim leaf bean: growing up in America. c. Phaseolus coccineus L. - scarlet runner: growing up in Spain, Guatemala and Mexico. d. Phaseolus filiformis Benth - slimjim bean: growing in the US Southwest and northern Mexico. e. Phaseolus lunatus L. - sicua bean: growing up in Argentina and America. f. Phaseolus macholatus Scheek - spotted bean: growing in Brazil. g. Phaseolus parvulus Greene - altos mountain pine bean: grows in Southeast Arizona. h. Phaseolus pedicellatus Benth - sonorant bean: grown in Mexico and Colombia. i. Phaseolus polymorphus S. Watson - bean variables: growth in North America and Mexico. Phaseolus polystachios (L.) Britton, Sterns &Poggenb. - Thicket bean: growing in the United States. k. Phaseolus ritensis M.E. Jones - santarita mountain bean: growing in the United States. l. Phaseolus vulgaris L. - kidney bean: grow evenly throughout the world.

2.2.2. Growing regions

Beans (Phaseolus vulgaris L.) are a widely cultivated vegetable crop in the world. This plant is not native to Indonesia but a primary origin is

19

Southern Mexico and Central America, while the secondary area is Peru, Ecuador, and Bolivia, and spread to Europe and Indonesia.[75]

Productivity and growth of beans are influenced by various factors climatic conditions of the environment are growing. Generally bean plants grown in the highlands of 1000 – 1500 m above sea level with a dry climate[76]and has been tested in the medium plateau 300-760m above sea level in South Tapanuli and can also grown in the low lands below 300m above sea level[77]and once planted 200-300m above sea level the result was satisfactory. The third medium depends on the type of varieties and types of growth. In order for optimum growth and yield of bean plants the average temperature needed 20-25°C, humidity 50-60%[77]and an average of 250-450 mm/month.[20] The type of soil suitable for growing beans are regosol and andosols ground contained in mountainous areas, requires oil pH5.5-6.0, crumbly texture with clay, sandy clay and clayey loam soil with an average temperature18-30°C. [20]

2.2.3. Morphology of plants

Bean shape usually bush or shrub and consists of two types growth, namely the type of vine growth (indeterminate) plant reaches a height of ± 2 m[77] even can reach 2.4 m and over 25 books flowering[78] and upright type / short (determinate) with a plant height of 30-50 cm)[77] with a slight amount of books and flowering formed at the tip of the main stem.[78]

Flowers of bean plants belonging perfect flower or androgynous (hermaphrodites), small size, long round shape (cylindrical) measuring ± 1 cm[77] and grows from young branches or young shoots are white, pink and purple. [79] Self-pollinated flowers with the help of the wind and insects. [78] There is a flat pod shape extending ± 20 cm wide, straight and short round ± 12 cm and a length of ± 15 cm round. Composition of segmented by the number of seed pods 5-14 / pods. The size and colour of the pods varies depending on the varieties. Seed size is rather large, oval shape and at the centre of the curved (concave), weight of 100 seeds from 16 to 40.6 grams of black.[20,77] Growth and production of component parts of bean plants varies according to the condition of each variety. Beans can be harvested at the age of 7-8 weeks after planting. [77]

2.2.4. Chemical ingredients

Bean plants have a variety of chemical constituents such as: folate, fibre, alkaloids, flavonoids, saponins, triterpenoida, steroid, stigmasterin, trigonelin, arginine, an amino acid, asparagine, kholina, tannins, fasin, starch, vitamin A, vitamin C and minerals (copper, magnesium, iron, potassium, calcium). [20,21]

2.2.5. Efficacy and Uses

Beans, which belong to the class of nuts, are foods that are rich sources of nutrients. Protective and therapeutic effects of substances contained in the beans have been widely investigated. The effects include: a decrease in serum cholesterol levels, improve many aspects of diabetes, and the metabolic benefits in weight control.[18]

Mackay, et al., (2002), conducted the research with the addition of 80 grams of beans in the daily diet for 6 weeks, obtained an increase in HDL cholesterol compared with no added beans in the diet.[80]

Several good effects that content of the beans:
2.2.5.1 Folate

Low levels off olic acid are associated with increased risk of coronary artery and cerebrovascular disease. In addition, 5,10-methylene tetra hydrofolate reductase mutation (MTHFR), which leads to reduced formation of 5-methyl tetra hydrofolate (5-MTHF, the active form of folate), has been reported to be a risk factor for vascular disease, which is also very dependent on folate levels. Administration of folic acid has been shown can improve endothelial function in hyperhomocysteinemia. Another study also found that administration of the active form of folic intra-arterial also can improve disturbance on endothelial function in patients with increased risk for atherosclerosis but have serum folate and homocysteine levels were normal.[81]

Folate allegedly involved in the regeneration of endogenous tetrahydrobiopterin (BH4), which is an important co factor for the formation NO. In addition, the antioxidant effects of folate can provide beneficial effects of endothelial function. Folic antioxidant effects may be direct or indirect, such as improvement of cellular antioxidant defence system. [81]

2.2.5.2 Fibre

Diets containing fibre has a great protective effect against atherosclerosis. Epidemiological data indicate that the intake of complex carbohydrates and fibre found in foods is inversely related to the incidence of coronary artery disease. Foods that contain fibre also slow the progression of atherosclerosis in animal models. Brown, et al., (2009), who conducted a meta-analysis of 67 studies on the effects of fibre on blood cholesterol levels, found that fibre intake significantly associated with a decrease in total cholesterol and LDL cholesterol. [18,82]

Fibre intake 3 grams per day can lower cholesterol levels approximately 5 mg / dl. When done estimation clinical studies on the treatment of cholesterol, it was found that the reduction of cholesterol by 5 mg / dl decrease the incidence of coronary artery disease approximately 4%.[82]

2.2.5.3 Flavonoids

Flavonoids belong to the group of natural substances with varying structures and phenols found in fruit, plants, grain, bark, roots, stems, flowers, tea, and wine. Over 4000 variations of flavonoids have been found, most of who play a role in giving colour to the flowers, fruits, and leaves. [83]

Flavonoids are known to have antioxidant effects that have a major role in the vascular system. Free radicals can oxidize LDL, which then can make the injury to the endothelial wall and subsequent role in the process of atherosclerosis. Arai, et al., (2000) found an inverse relationship between intake of flavonoids and total plasma cholesterol concentrations. [84]

Compounds of flavonoids such as phenolhydroxylation C3-C6 units in the chain of the aromaticring. Flavonoids are known for having an anti-oxidant that protects the body from reactive oxygen species (ROS). Free radicals can cause damage to the cell membrane. Anti-oxidant defence mechanisms in the body involve several enzymes such as superoxide dismutase, catalase, and glutathione peroxidase. Increased production of ROS cause injury and produce consumption and depletion of endogenous scavenging compounds. Flavonoids have an addictive effect of endogenous scavenging compounds. [83,85]

Because it has the effect of anti-oxidants, flavonoids also have an effect on the vascular system. Several studies have found that flavonoids may protect against coronary heart disease. Hertog et al found that flavonoids consumed from the diet can reduce the risk of death from coronary heart disease in older aged patients. [84]

Several studies in humans and animals have found that flavonoids have an important role in the prevention of cognitive impairment associated with aging, decreased motor, mood, and the prevention of oxidative stress such as cerebral ischemia. [86-91] The exact mechanism of how flavonoids work as a neuroprotective in vivo is not known fully. [92]

In addition to the effects anti sclerosis, flavonoids also have anti-inflammatory, anti-tumor, anti-thrombogenic, anti-osteoporosis, and anti-viral (Figure 3). [83,93]

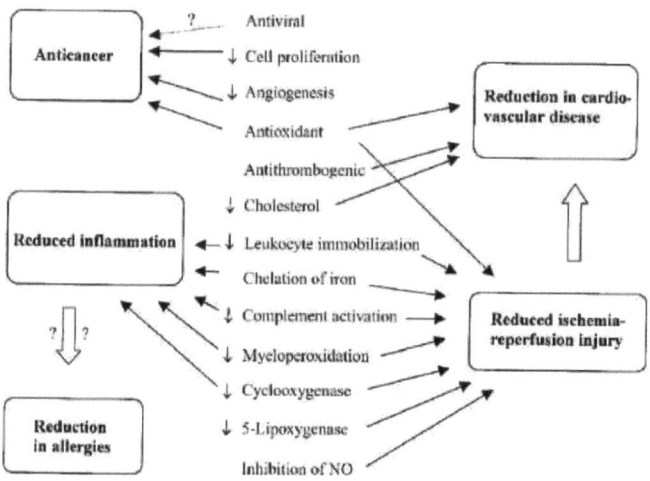

Figure 3. Hypothesis on Mechanism of Flavonoids and Their Effects on Disease[83]

2.2.5.4 Saponins

Malinow, et al., have been doing research with saponin administration in monkeys and found a decrease in serum cholesterol levels. This occurs due to the decrease in intestinal cholesterol absorption, increased excretion of endogenous and exogenous steroids through faecal.[94]

2.2.5.5 Vitamin A

Vitamin A supplementation can reduce total cholesterol levels in rats. Jeyakumar, et al., (2007), who conducted the study found that the decline is associated with over expression of SR-BI m RNA. SR-BI is a scavenger receptor class BI involved in the regulation of HDL cholesterol through the RCT (Reverse Cholesterol Transport), cardioprotection, steroidogenesis, and reproduction.[95]

2.3 Hypothesis Research:

2.3.1 Hypothesis major

Bean extract can affect the plasma levels of LDL and oxidized LDL in subjects carriers of LOX-1 gene polymorphisms 3'UTR188C / T.

2.3.2 Hypothesis minor

a. There are differences between the mean plasma levels of LDL and oxidized LDL with a carrier subject LOX-1 gene polymorphisms 3'UTR188C / T.

b. There are differences in mean changes in plasma levels of LDL and oxidized LDL in the group given bean extract with control

CHAPTER III
RESEARCH METHODOLOGY

3.1 Material and Methods

This study is true randomized experiment with a pre test – post test design with control group

3.2 Subjects

Subjects were paramedics at Putri Hijau Hospital, Medan. 40 participants were recruited with inclusion criteria: 1. Normal subjects both men and women aged 30-50 years. 2. Have a complete personal data such as name, address, age, and phone number, or mobile phones. 3. Willing to participate in the study and signed a consent form after getting a description of the study (informed consent). Exclusion criteria: 1. Suffering hypertension, diabetes mellitus (DM), and impaired renal function 2. Intolerance to nuts. Drop out criteria: 1. If during the period of the study subjects died or refused to continue the research. 2. If during the study subjects did not consume bean extract that has been established or suffering severe illness.

3.3 Treatment

Subjects underwent pre treatment for one week (baseline period, starting from H – 6 to day 0), with dietary habits such as usual and asked not to consume any kind of food that comes from the nuts.

On day 0, patients underwent blood sampling for examination LDL, Ox-LDL levels and LOX-1 gene polymorphism 3'UTR188CT. Subjects get an explanation about the dosage and how to take the extract.

Treatments from day 0, subjects were divided into four groups. The first group (A) consumed beans every day as much as 40 grams per day were made in the capsule, the second group (B) 80 grams, the third group (C) 120 grams, while the fourth group (D) taking placebo. Consumption schedule is while eating. Subjects will also call or send short messages service/SMS via mobile phone to remind drinking extract schedule.

3.4 Blood test

Blood samples (Whole Blood) is taken when the study participants were in fasting 10-12 hours using a 10 cc syringe already containing anticoagulant (heparin) on the vein by a trained nurse. The blood sample is then sent to a laboratory for examination of LDL (Multigent Architect), Ox-LDL levels[96] and LOX-1 gene polymorphism 3'UTR188CT (PCR - RFLP method).[97]

3.5 Statistical analysis

LDL and Ox-LDL level data were normally distributed. To evaluate effect of bean extract to LDL and Ox-LDL level were compared with unpaired t-test. To evaluate difference of Ox-LDL level on LOX-1 gene polymorphism 3'UTR188CT using ANOVA. We considered a value of $p < 0.05$ as significant. Data analyses were performed by using SPSS 16.0.

CHAPTER IV
RESULTS

4.1 Phytochemical test results

Plants are used as research materials are beans planted in Berastagi City, Karo, Sumatera Utara Province. The bean plants grown using organic fertilizers and harvested after that is old enough for 6 weeks. Beans are then selected which are not eaten by pests.

The result of phytochemical screening of the bean is known that beans contain chemical compounds as shown in Table1.

Table1.Results of phytochemical screening bulbs beans

No	Examination	Results
1	Alkaloida	+
2	Saponin	+
3	Tanin	-
4	Flavonoid	+
5	Triterpenoid/steroid	+
6	Glikosida	+

Description: +(Positive) =Contains classes of compounds

- (Negative) = Not Contains classes of compounds

Bean extract screening results indicate that the beans contain flavonoid chemical compounds which have generally been known to act as an antioxidant that is as free radical catcher because it contains hydroxyl groups. Free radicals can oxidize LDL, which then can make the injury to the endothelial wall and subsequent role in the process of atherosclerosis. In addition to the effects anti sclerosis, flavonoids also have anti-inflammatory, anti-tumor, anti-thrombogenic, anti-osteoporosis, and anti-viral effects.

Flavonoids in crude drug powder and ethanol extract can be aglycones and glycosides. Aglycone generally has antioxidant activity and radical catcher higher than flavonoid glycosides, flavonoids glycosides because the phenolic hydroxy group is an active group of antioxidants and radical catchers have binding force of sugar. The presence of a phenolic hydroxyl group can capture free radicals.

4.2. Tes teffect of extract beans on LDL and Oxidized LDL levels in plasma LOX-1 Polymorphisms3'UTR 188 C/T

4.2.1. General characteristics of the study subjects.

Research conducted at the Laboratory of Clinical Research Prodia Medan and Jakarta, the Eijkman Institute in Jakarta and Putri Hijau Hospital Medan since November 2012 - July 2013 by selecting a random sample. Samples taken as many as 40 subjects consisting of men were 12 subjects (30%) and women totalling 28 subjects (70%).

All subjects were divided into 4 groups, each consisting of 10 subjects, namely group A (which is given bean extract 40 g/day), group B (80 g/day), group C (120 g/day), and group D (placebo). On the seventh day, the rest of the capsule had count and obtained five study participants did not consume capsules as has been suggested so that later the participants were excluded from the study (drop out). The fifth subject is derived from one subject group A, group C 3 subjects and group D 1 subject, bringing the total study participants who completed the study of 35subjects, as shown in Scheme1.

Group A (40 g/day) Group B (80 g/day) Group C (120 g/ day) Group D (Plasebo)

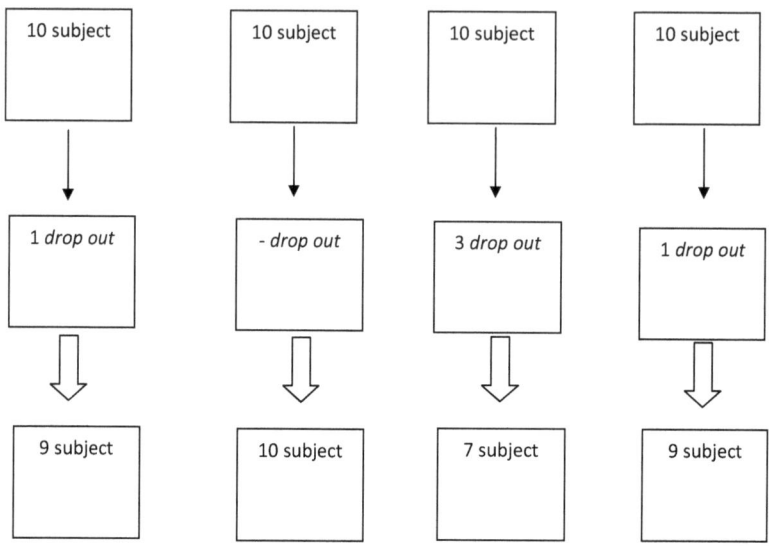

Scheme1.The research sample

Of the 35 subjects, most subjects were women 27 subjects (77%) and men 8 subjects (23%). The baseline characteristics of the subjects by study group can be seen in Table 2.

Table 2. The baseline characteristics of the subjects by study group

Characteristic	Bean extract 40 g (N=9)	Bean extract 80 g (N=10)	Bean extract 120 g (N=7)	Placebo (N=9)
Sex female – no (%)	7 (78)	8 (80)	6 (86)	6 (67)
Old - years	$43 \pm 4,6^{*}$	$38,2 \pm 5,3^{**}$	$44,43 \pm 4,6^{***}$	$38,78 \pm 5,2$
Blood sugar	$87 \pm 8,7$	$87,7 \pm 8,2$	$80 \pm 7,6$	$86,78 \pm 7$
Ureum	$20,89 \pm 5,6$	$20,8 \pm 5,6$	$19,43 \pm 2,4$	$18,22 \pm 4,6$
Creatinin	$0,84 \pm 0,26$	$0,81 \pm 0,26$	$0,76 \pm 0,16$	$0,83 \pm 0,18$
Hypertension – no (%)	-	-	-	-
Dyslipidaemia – no (%)	6 (67)	5 (50)	4 (57)	3 (33)

* $p<0.05$ compared to extract 80 g

** $p<0.05$ compared to extract 40 g and 120 g

*** $p<0.05$ compared to extract 80 g and placebo

From the above table it can be seen that the only significant difference was age between subjects who consumed the extract 40 g/day to 80 g/day, 80 g/day to 120 g/day and between 120 g/day with placebo.

Participants were observed for 14 days. Most complaints of participants during eating bean extract is digestive disorders such as heartburn, nausea, and abdominal discomfort as many as six participants (17%), followed by squash as many as three participants (9%) and headache 1 participants (3%).

4.2.2 Test LOX-1 gene polymorphism 3'UTR188 C/T

Test LOX-1 gene polymorphism 3'UTR188 C/T conducted at the Eijkman Institute in Jakarta. From 35 subjects examined LOX-1 gene polymorphisms tha thave gained 3'UTR188 C/T CC genotype as many as15 subjects (43%), CT 17 subjects (49%), and TT 3 subjects (8%). Test results of LOX-1 gene polymorphism 3'UTR188 C/T based study group can be seen in the figure 4 below.

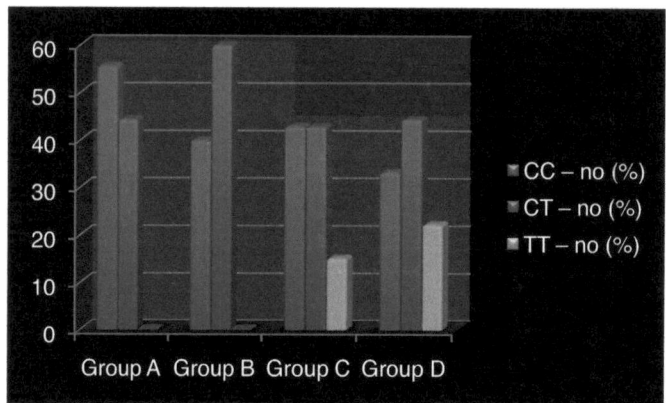

Figure 4.Test results LOX-1 gene polymorphism 3'UTR188 C/T based on the study group

From 35 subjects who had a C allele were 47 (67%) and T alleles were 23 (33%) that can be seen in the figure 5 below.

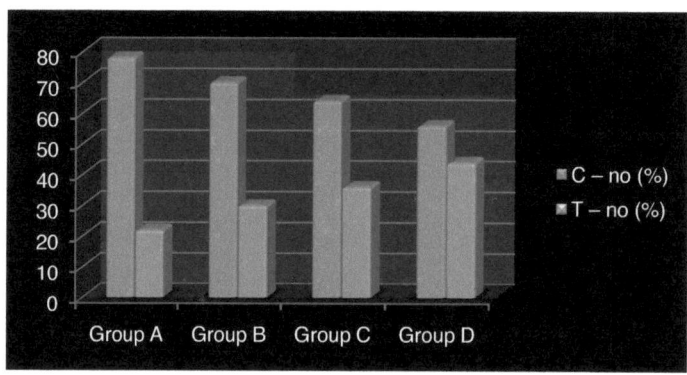

Figure 5. Frequency of alleles based study group

From figure 5, it can be seen that the C allele had a greater frequency than T allele in all groups.

4.2.3 Levels of oxidized LDL plasma

TT genotype had higher levels of Ox-LDL plasma than other genotypes both before and after treatment that can be seen in the table below.

Table 3. Ox-LDL plasma levels before treatment based on gene polymorphisms LOX-1 3'UTR188CT

Parameter	N	Ox-LDL	p
CC	15	39.9 ± 19.4	
CT	17	42,8 ± 61,2	0.648
TT	3	49,9 ± 8,3	

Table 4. Ox-LDL plasma levels after treatment based on gene polymorphisms LOX-1 3'UTR188CT

Parameter	N	Ox-LDL	p
CC	15	55.93 ± 12.6	
CT	17	53.9 ± 10.3	0.630
TT	3	60.3 ± 5.7	

When compared LDL and Ox-LDL plasma level before and after treatment, the results can be seen in the figure 6 below.

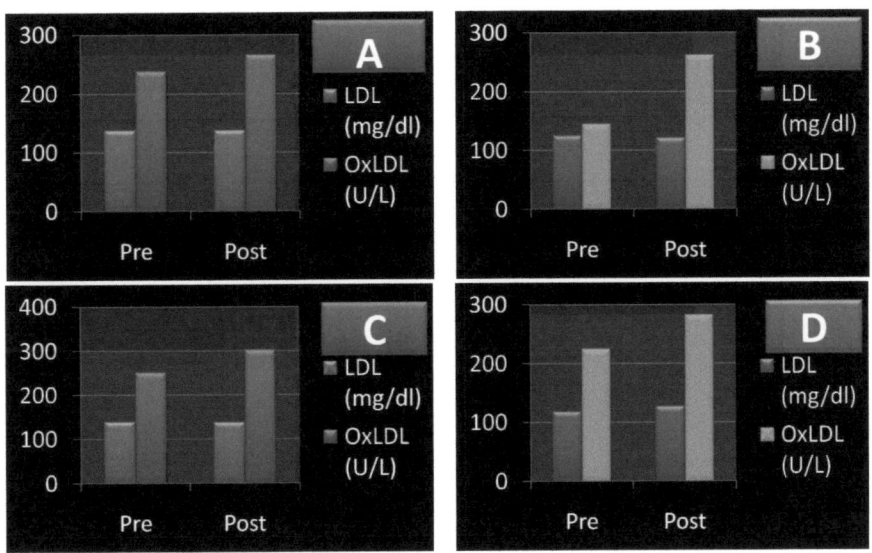

Figure 6. LDL and oxidized LDL levels before and after treatment

From figure 6, it can be seen that the LDL cholesterol decreased in all group gave extract, although not significantly. In group B and group C found increased plasma Ox-LDL were significant after treatment.

CHAPTER V
DISCUSSION

In the last three decades, large studies have shown that oxidized LDL is a useful marker for cardiovascular disease. High levels of oxidized LDL are associated with the presence of some disturbances in tissue vascularisation and show that oxidized LDL is a potential prognostic marker for early detection of health problems in the future. Oxidized LDL induces multiple effects of pro atherosclerotic, including activation of endothelial and smooth muscle proliferation. Increased plasma levels of oxidized LDL found in patients with pathological conditions such as cardiovascular disease, cerebral infarction, and patients with chronic kidney disease who undergo haemodialysis.[49,55,98-101]

Known active compounds contained in crude drugs facilitate the choice of solvent and appropriate extraction method. To achieve a desired extract, it must be met quality standards extract material that cannot be separated from process control. Standard process can guarantee a standardized product. Based on the above, the manufacture of bean extract has met standardization conducted in the Laboratory of Traditional Medicine Faculty of Pharmacy, University of Sumatra Utara, Indonesia.

Results phytochemical screening of beans simplicia that are extracted by using ethanol 70% identified containing the compound such as alkaloids, saponins, flavonoids, triterpenoids/steroids, and glycosides. This phytochemical test results indicate that extract of beans do not contain some material that is owned by the bean itself lik efolate, fibre, arginine, an aminoacid, asparagine, kholina, tannins, fasin, starch, vitamin A, vitamin C, and minerals(copper, magnesium, iron, potassium, calcium).

Results of test polymorphism gen 3'UTR188 C/T found most genotypes in this study is the CT was 49%, followed by CC 43%, and TT as much as 8%. These results are consistent with studies conducted by Sentinelli, et al were also found most is the CT genotype, followed by CC, and TT. While the research conducted by Kurnaz et al, found most is the CT genotype, followed by TT, and CC genotype. [13-102]

This study find initial plasma oxidized LDL levels in group B (participants who received bean extract 80 g/day) is lower than the other groups significantly, while the initial plasma oxidized LDL levels in group C (participants who received bean extract 120 g/day) is higher than another group was significantly mainly from group B. After treatment found increased levels of plasma oxidized LDL in each group although the differences were not significant.

This study found a decrease in levels of LDL cholesterol in the group given bean extract with a greater reduction occurred in the group given bean extract 80 g / day, although not significantly. While plasma oxidized LDL levels found an increase in all groups, whereas in the group given bean extract 80 and 120 g / day found a significant difference.

Overall, results of this study found no change in plasma oxidized LDL levels as expected. There are some reason that may underlie this, like content of bean extract not as complete as content of materials or substances contained in the bean itself, such as fibre. Meta-analysis conducted by Brown et al, found that water-soluble fibre can significantly reduce total cholesterol and LDL. The mechanism of fibre can lowering cholesterol include: bonding fibres with intra-luminal cholesterol during formation, inhibit the formation of hepatic fatty acid with production of short chain fatty acids such as acetate, butyrate, and propionate, alter intestinal motility smooth, slow down the absorption of macronutrients, causing an increase in insulin sensitivity and increase satiety so overall reduces input. [82] In addition to fibre, a substance that also contributes to lowering cholesterol that is not contained in the extract is folat, and vitamin A.

Another possibility to increase the levels of oxidized LDL after consuming bean extract is antioxidant that is found in the bean extract does not contain sufficient antioxidant activity. It is also delivered by Silaste, et al (2004), who conducted the research with giving low fat diet, low vegetable, and low-fat diet, high vegetable found an increase in oxidized LDL by 27% and! 9% sequentially. Another possibility is that because it is not clear how the oxidation of LDL occurs in vivo, human trials using anti-oxidants may be incorrect.[103]

Several animal studies show dietary supplements with anti-oxidants substances such as Probucol, vitamin E, coenzymes Q, diphenylphenylenediamine or butylatedhydroxy toluene can accelerate the development of atherosclerosis. [55] In humans, dietary with antioxidant supplements have not shown evidence of success as protective. Large-scale clinical trials in humans showed overall, supplementation with vitamin E, beta carotene, or a combination of several anti-oxidants cannot lower the risk of coronary artery disease.[104-106]

Large clinical trials of the anti-oxidants, mostly using vitamin E and beta carotene, did not give satisfactory results. Meta analysis of the study data showed no benefit with the use of anti-oxidants on the outcome of cardiovascular events. [107,108] Another clinical trial to approximately 40,000 healthy women who were followed for 10 years shows that consumed high doses of vitamin E cannot reduce the incidence of cardiovascular disorders.[109] There are several possibilities for this test fails to provide a satisfactory effect although oxidative modification is an important element in the pathogenesis of human disease that also previously shown in animal experiments. The possibility for example, vitamin E may be an anti-oxidant that is not appropriate in humans, the dose given is too small. It is important also is possible the giving of anti-oxidants assessed late, giving of anti-oxidants may be useful only in certain patients, such as patients who are exposed more to oxidative stress. So overall, it can be hypothesized that not all anti-oxidants, not at all doses, and not at all an individual provide useful results. Based on existing data it is not advisable to use an anti-oxidant supplements for the prevention and treatment of cardiovascular disease.[110-113]The same thing may happen to anti-oxidants contained in the bean extract.

Initial hypothesis indicates that oxidative modification plays an important role in the pathogenesis of atherosclerosis in most individuals. But based on the above hypothesis oxidative modification may have a role in individuals with substantial oxidative stress, such as individuals with renal failure undergoing haemodialysis or diabetes mellitus.[114,115]

The results of this study also found reduction in LDL cholesterol in all groups was given extracts beans, but occur increase in plasma levels of oxidized LDL. This suggests that although LDL cholesterol can be lowered but not automatically plasma oxidized LDL levels go down as well. These results are also consistent with research conducted by Fang, et al., (2011) who conducted the research to find the relationship between plasma oxidized LDL and carotid plaque in the Han ethnic group in China. The results of this study found that although the group had plaques have lower LDL levels than non-plaque group but that group had higher levels of oxidized LDL plaque which was significantly higher than non-plaque group. Studies conducted Silaste et al, also found a decrease in LDL by study participants who consumed a diet low in fat and high in vegetables but have higher levels of oxidized LDL compared to baseline.[103,116] The relationship between the levels of oxidized LDL with cardiovascular risk factors not yet fully understood. Oxidized LDL were found in the walls of blood vessels more than that found in plasma.[117,118]

An increased plasma level of oxidized LDL is also known to be temporary. Naruko, et al., (2006) reported an increase in plasma levels of oxidized LDL in patients with acute myocardial infarction approximately 3.5

times compared to normal subjects. But increased levels of plasma oxidized LDL is then dropped to near normal when the patient is discharged from the hospital. The same result was obtained by Uno et al., (2003) who observed plasma levels of oxidized LDL in patients with cerebral infarction. Plasma oxidized LDL levels of patients with cerebral infarction increased on the first day of the disease and then returned to the normal range within 30 days.[100,119]

This study also found that in group A, those with the CC genotype had higher levels of oxidized LDL than those with genotype CT both before and after administration of bean extract 40 g / day. Whereas in group B, the participants with the CC genotype had higher levels of oxidized LDL than those with genotype CT before administration bean extract, but after giving bean extract 80 g / day participants with CT genotype had higher levels of oxidized LDL than those with the CC genotype. In group C participants with CT genotype had higher levels of oxidized LDL than those with genotype TT and CC before bean extract, but after administration bean extract 120 g / day, participants with the TT genotype had higher levels of oxidized LDL than those with genotype CT and CC. In the placebo group, participants with CT genotype had higher levels of oxidized LDL than those with the TT and CC genotype both before and after treatment.

The results of this study also found that participants with CT and TT genotypes had higher levels of oxidized LDL than those with the CC genotype. As was explained earlier, oxidized LDL levels would be elevated in patients with cardiovascular disorders, so that participants with CT and TT genotypes have the possibility for the occurrence of cardiovascular disorders higher than the other genotypes. This is consistent with studies conducted by Mango, et al., (2003) in which it was found that participants with genotype TT or CT have a greater risk for the development of acute myocardial infarction.[16,120,121]

CHAPTER VI
CONCLUSIONS AND RECOMMENDATIONS

6.1 Conclusions

Based on research results, it can be concluded several things:

A. General Conclusions

Standardized bean extract containing active compounds such as alkaloids, saponins, flavonoids, triterpenoids/steroids, and glycosides have the effect of lowering plasma LDL levels in subjects treated but also may increase the plasma levels of oxidized LDL on that subject.

B. Special Conclusion

1. Test phytochemical extracts of beans

Result of phytochemical screening, bean extract contains several compounds like alkaloids, saponins, flavonoids, triterpenoids/steroids, and glycosides.

2. Test bean extract effect on plasma levels of LDL and oxidized LDL and its relation with LOX-1 gene polymorphisms 3'UTR188 C/T.

a. Test LOX-1 gene polymorphism 3'UTR188 C/T.

This study found most of the study participants genotype is a heterozygous genotype (CT) followed by a homozygous genotype (CC).

b. Plasma levels of LDL and oxidized LDL

This study found after administration bean extract found reduction of plasma LDL levels with the largest decrease was in the group given bean extract 80 g/day, followed by the given bean extract 120 g/day and 40 g/day.

This study also found an increase in plasma oxidized LDL levels after administration bean extract with the highest increase was in the group given bean extract 80 g/day, followed by the given bean extract 120 g/day and 40 g/day.

c. Plasma oxidized LDL levels by genotype

This study found that participants with CT and TT genotypes had higher levels of plasma oxidized LDL than those with the CC genotype.

6.2 Advice

1. Research effects of extracts bean (Phaseolus vulgaris L) on the levels of LDL and oxidized LDL and its relation with LOX-1 gene polymorphisms 3'UTR188 C / T as a preventive measure risk of atherosclerosis is a preliminary study on the efficacy of bean extract on plasma LDL and oxidized LDL that had never done.
2. Because not all materials or substances contained in the beans also contained in the extract, it is advisable to conduct research directly to the bean itself.
3. Need to do further studies on the isolation and fraction level of the substances contained in the extract beans of the plasma levels of LDL and oxidized LDL
4. It should be further evaluated for anti-oxidants which may have a beneficial effect by lowering the levels of oxidized LDL.
5. Because there is no standard of plasma oxidized LDL examination procedure, it is advisable to conduct research using a different procedure with the procedure used for this study.
6. Because found temporal changes in plasma oxidized LDL levels, it is advisable also to do some research of plasma oxidized LDL levels serially to see the changes.

REFERENCES

1. Miettinen, TA, Railo, M, Lepantalo, M, Gylling, H, 2005. Plant sterols in serum and in atherosclerotic plaques of patients undergoing endarterectomy. J Am CollCardiol, vol. 45, pp. 1794-801

2. Falk, E, Fuster, V, 2006. Atherogenesis and its determinants. In: Hurst's The Heart. Fuster V, Alexander RW, O'Rourke RA, eds. 11thed. New York. McGraw-Hill, pp, 1065-94.

3. Fraley, AE, Tsimikas, S, 2006. Clinical applications of circulating oxidized low-density lipoprotein biomarkers in cardiovascular disease. Curr Opin Lipidol, vol. 17, pp. 502–9

4. Steinberg D, 2002. Atherogenesis in perspective: hypercholesterolemia and inflammation as partners in crime. Nat Med, vol. 8, pp. 1211–7.

5. Libby, P, 2005. Act local, act global: Inflammation and the multiplicity of "vulnerable" coronary plaques. J Am Coll Cardiol, vol. 45, pp. 1600–2

6. Heinecke, JW, 2006. Lipoprotein oxidation in cardiovascular disease: chief culprit or innocent bystander? NJEM, vol. 203, no. 4, pp. 813–6.

7. Basic Health Research, 2013. Badan Penelitian dan Pengembangan Kesehatan Menteri Kesehatan RI, pp. 92.

8. Anderson, JW, Major, AW, 2004. Pulses and lipaemia, short- and long-term effect: Potential in the prevention of cardiovascular disease. British Journal of Nutrition, vol. 88, Suppl 3, pp. S263-S71

9. Holvoet, P, Kritchevsky, SB, Tracy, RP, 2004. The metabolic syndrome, circulating oxidized LDL, and risk of myocardial infarction in well functioning elderly people in the health, aging, and body composition cohort. Diabetes, vol. 53, pp. 1068–73

10. Verreth W, De Keyzer D, Pelat M, 2004. Weight loss associated induction of peroxisome proliferator activated receptor-alpha and peroxisome proliferator activated receptor-γ correlate with reduced

atherosclerosis and improved cardiovascular function in obese insulin-resistant mice. Circulation, vol. 110(20), pp. 3259–69

11. Packard, RS, Libby, P, 2008. Inflammation in atherosclerosis; from vascular biology to biomarker discovery and risk prediction. Clinical Chemistry, vol. 54, pp. 24-31

12. Dunn, S, Vohra, RS, Murphy, JE, Vanniasinkam, SH, Walker, JH, Ponnambalam, S, 2008. The lectin-like oxidized low-density-lipoprotein receptor: a pro-inflammatory factor in vascular disease. Biochem J, vol. 409, pp. 349-55.

13. Kurnaz, O, Teker, ABA, Aydogan, HY, Tekeli, A, Isbir, T, 2011. The LOX-1 3'UTR188 CT polymorphism and coronary artery disease in Turkish patients. Mol Biol Rep : DOI 10.1007/s11033-011-1222-3

14. Sawamura T, Kume N, Aoyama T, Moriwaki H, Hoshikawa H, Aiba Y, *et al*, 2007. An endothelial receptor for oxidized low-density lipoprotein. Nature, vol. 403, pp. 73–7.

15. Yoshimoto, R, Fujita, Y, Iwamoto, AK, Takaya, T, Sawamura, T, 2011. The Discovery of LOX-1, its Ligands and Clinical Significance. Cardiovasc Drugs Ther. vol. 25. pp. 379–91.

16. Mango, R, Clementi, F, Borgaini, P, Forleo, GB, Federici, M, Contino, G, *et al*, 2003. Association of single nucleotide polymorphisms in the oxidised LDL receptor 1 (OLR1) gene in patients with acute myocardial infarction. J Med Genet, vol. 40, pp. 933-6

17. Chen Q, Reis SE, Kammerer C, Craig, WY, LaPierre SE, Zimmer, EL, *et al*, 2003. Genetic variation in lectin-like oxidized low-density lipoprotein receptor 1 (LOX1) gene and the risk of coronary artery disease. Circulation, vol. 107, pp. 3146-51

18. Anderson, JW, Smith, BM, Washnock, CS, 2009. Cardiovascular and renal benefits of dry bean and soybean intake. Am J ClinNutr, vol. 78 (suppl), pp. 464S-74S

19. Lovegrove, JA, Clohessy, A, Milon, H, Williams, CM, 2000. Modest doses of b-glucan do not reduce concentrations of potentially atherogenic lipoproteins. Am J ClinNutr, vol. 72, pp 49–55.

20. Science and Technoogy Information Centre, 2008. Buncis. http://www.iptek.net.id/ind/teknologi_Pangan/index.php?mnu=2&id=298 . Hal: 1-5

21. Kabagambe, EK, Baylin, A, Narvarez, ER, Siles, X, Campos, H, 2005. Decreased consumption of dried mature beans is positively associated with urbanization and nonfatal acute myocardial infarction. J Nutr, vol. 135, pp. 1770-5.

22. Hansen D, 2005. Plant sterols in beans. Available at: http://www.ehow.com>>drugs& supplements

23. Ross, R, 2006. The pathogenesis of atherosclerosis: an update. N Engl J Med, vol. 353, pp. 488 –500.

24. Ross, R, 2009. Atherosclerosis – an inflammatory disease. N Engl J Med, vol. 357, pp. 115-26

25. Pirillo, A, Norata, GD, Catapano, AL, 2013. LOX-1, Ox-LDL, and Atherosclerosis. Mediators of Inflammation, vol. 2013, pp. 1-13.

26. Libby, P, 2012. Inflammation and atherosclerosis. Arteriosclerosis, Thrombosis, and Vascular Biology, vol. 32, no. 9, pp. 2045-51.

27. Hansson, GK, Libby, P, 2006. The immune response in atherosclerosis: a double-edged sword. Nat Rev Immunol, vol. 6, pp. 508 –19.

28. Ehara, S, Ueda, M, Naruko, T, et al, 2007. Elevated levels of oxidized low density lipoprotein show a positive relationship with the severity of acute coronary syndrome .Circulation , vol. 110, no. 15, pp. 1955-60.

29. Itabe, H, Takano, T, 2000. Oxidized Low Density Lipoprotein : The Occurrence and Metabolism in Circulation and in Foam Cells. Journal of Atherosclerosis and Thrombosis, vol. 7, pp. 123-131.

30. Shoenfeld, Y, Harats, D, Wick, G, 2004. Atherosclerosis and Autoimmunity Amsterdam: Elsevier; 1–370

31. Shoenfeld, Y, Wu, R, Dearing, LD, Matsuura, E, 2004. Are Anti–Oxidized Low-Density Lipoprotein Antibodies Pathogenic or Protective?Circulation,.vol. 110, pp. 2552-8.

32. Ross, R, 2008. The pathogenesis of atherosclerosis: a perspective for the 1990s,. Nature, vol. 402, pp. 801–9.

33. Virella, MF, Virella, G, 2013. Pathogenic Role of Modified LDL Antibodies and Immune Complexes in Atherosclerosis. J Artheroscler Thromb, vol. 20, pp. 1-12.

34. Lundberg, AM, Hansson, GK, 2010. Innate immune signals in atherosclerosis. Clin Immunol, vol. 134, pp. 5-24.

35. Andersson, J, Libby, P, Hansson, GK, 2010. Adaptive immunity and atherosclerosis. Clin Immunol, vol. 134, pp. 33-46.

36. Virella, MF, Virella, G, 2010. Clinical significance of the humoral immune response to modified LDL. Clin Immunol, vol. 134, pp. 55-65.

37. Grundy, SM, Cleeman, JI, Merz, CNB, Brewer, HB, Clark LT &Hunninghake, DB, 2004, Implications of Recent Clinical Trial for the National Cholesterol Education Program Adult Treatment Panel III Guidelines. Circulation, vol. 110, pp. 227-39.

38. Miettinen, H, Lehto, S, Salomaa, V, Mahonen, M, Niemela, M, Haffner, SM, 2007. Impact of diabetes on mortality after the first myocardial infarction. Diabetes Care, vol. 44, pp. 69-75.

39. National Cholesterol Education Program (NCEP) Expert Panel on Detection, Evaluation, and Treatment of High Blood Cholesterol in Adults (Adult Treatment Panel III) 2002. Third Report of the National Cholesterol Education Program (NCEP) Expert Panel on Detection, Evaluation, and Treatment of High Blood Cholesterol in Adults (Adult Treatment Panel III) final report. Circulation, vol. 106, pp. 3143-421.

40. Pyorala, K, De Backer, G, Graham, I, Poole-Wilson, P, 2004. Prevention of coronary heart disease in clinical practice. Atherosclerosis, vol. 163, pp. 121-61.

41. Hoogen, PCW, Feskens, EJM, Nagelkerke, NJD, Menotti, A, Nissinen, A, Kromhout, D, 2004. The relation between blood pressure and mortality due to coronary heart disease among men in different parts of world. N Engl J Med, vol, 350, pp. 1-8.

42. Wilson, PWF, D'Agostino, RB, Levy, D, Belanger, AM, Silbershatz, H, Kannel, WB, 2008. Prediction of coronary heart disease using risk factor categories. Circulation, vol. 113, pp. 1837-47.

43. Tsimikas, S, Glass, C, Steinberg, D, *et al,* 2004. Lipoproteins, lipoprotein oxidation and atherogenesis. In: Chien KR, editor. Molecular basis of cardiovascular disease: A companion to Braunwald's heart disease. Philadelphia: W.B. Saunders Company, pp. 385–413

44. Holvoet, P, Perez, G, Zhao, Z, 2006. Malondialdehyde-modified low density lipoproteins in patients with atherosclerotic disease. J Clin Invest, vol. 114, pp. 2611–9

45. Horkko, S, Bird, DA, Miller E, 2007. Monoclonal autoantibodies specific for oxidized phospholipids or oxidized phospholipid-protein adducts inhibit macrophage uptake of oxidized low-density lipoproteins. J Clin Invest, vol. 109, pp. 117–28

46. Itabe, H, Yamamoto, H, Imanaka T, 2009. Sensitive detection of oxidatively modified low density lipoprotein using a monoclonal antibody. J Lipid Res, vol. 44, pp. 45–53.

47. Tomkin, GH, Owens, D, 2012. LDL as a Cause of Atherosclerosis. The Open Atherosclerosis & Thrombosis Journal, vol.5, pp. 13-21

48. Heart Protection Study Collaborative Group, 2002. MRC/BHF Heart Protection Study of cholesterol lowering with simvastatin in 20,536 high-risk individuals: a randomised placebo-controlled trial. Lancet, vol. 360 no. 9326, pp. 7-22.

49. Levitan, I, Volkov, S, Subbaiah, PV, 2010. Oxidized LDL : diversity, patterns of recognition, and pathophysiology. Antioxidants, and Redox Signaling, vol. 132, no. 1, pp. 39-75.

50. Hayashida, K, Kume, N, Murase, T, Minami M, Nakagawa, D, Inada, T, *et al*, 2005. Serum soluble lectin-like oxidized low-density lipoprotein receptor-1 levels are elevated in acute coronary syndrome : a novel marker for early diagnosis. Circulation, vol. 112, pp. 812-8.

51. Sämpi, M, Ukkola, O, Päivänsalo, M, Kesäniemi, A, Binder, CJ, Hörkkö, S, 2008. Plasma Interleukin-5 Levels Are Related to Antibodies Binding to Oxidized Low-Density Lipoprotein and to Decreased Subclinical Atherosclerosis. JACC, vol. 52, no. 17, pp. 1370-8.

52. Hansson, GK, 2005. Inflammation, atherosclerosis, and coronary artery disease. N Engl J Med, vol. 352, pp. 1685–95.

53. Binder, CJ, Chang, MK, Shaw, PX, 2002. Innate and acquired immunity in atherogenesis. Nat Med, vol. 8, pp. 1218 –26

54. Zhang, Y. Dawson, VL, Dawson, TM, 2000. Oxidative stress and genetics in the pathogenesis of Parkinson's disease. Neurobiol. Dis, vol. 7, pp. 240-50.

55. Witztum, JL, Steinberg, D, 2001. The oxidative modification hypothesis of atherosclerosis: does it hold for humans?. Trends Cardiovasc Med, vol. 11, pp. 93-102.

56. Witztum, JL, Steinberg, D, 2004. Role of oxidized low density lipoprotein in atherogenesis. J Clin Invest, vol. 96, pp. 1785-92.

57. Tsimikas, S, Witztum, JL, 2001. Measuring circulating oxidized low density lipoprotein to evaluate coronary risk. Circulation, vol. 103, pp. 1930-2.

58. Vaatrala, O, 2010. Antibodies to oxidized LDL. Lupus, vol. 16, pp. 202-5

59. Ronchini, KROM, Goto, H, Duarte, AJS, Gidlund, M, 2013. Anti-Oxidized LDL Antibodies as Atherosclerosis Development Markers in HIV Patients Undergoing Antiretroviral Therapy: A Longitudinal Cohort Study. International Trends In Immunity, vol.1, pp. 72-8.

60. Barbaro, G, 2006. Highly active antiretroviral therapy-associated metabolic syndrome: pathogenesis and cardiovascular risk. Am. J. Ther, vol. 13, no. 3, pp. 248-60.

61. Iglesias, A, Bots, ML, Grobbee, DE, Hofman, A, Witteman, JC, 2004. Carotid intima-media thickness at different sites: relation to incident myocardial infarction; The Rotterdam Study. Eur Heart J, vol. 31, no. 12, pp. 934-40.

62. Navarra, T, Turco, SD, Berti, S, Basta, G, 2010. The Lectin-Like Oxidized Low- Density Lipoprotein Receptor-1 and Its Soluble Form: Cardiovascular Implications. J AtherosclerThromb, vol. 17, pp. 317-31.

63. Berliner, JA, Heinecke, JW, 2006. The role of oxidized lipoprotein in atherogenesis. Free RadicBiol Med, vol. 27, pp. 707-27.

64. Oberley, TD, 2002. Oxidative damage and cancer. Am J Pathol, vol. 160, pp. 403-8.

65. Reiss, AB, Anwar, K, Wirkowski, P, 2009. Lectin-Like Oxidized Low Density Lipoprotein Receptor 1 (LOX-1) in Atherogenesis: A Brief Review. Curr Med Chem, vol. 16, pp. 2641-52

66. Droge, W, 2008. Free radicals in the physiological control of cell function. Physiol Rev, vol. 89, pp. 47-95.

67. Tezel, G, 2007. Oxidative stress in glaucomatous neurodegeneration: Mechanisms and Consequences. Prog Retin Eye Res, vol. 25, no. 5, pp. 490-513.

68. Ferreira, SM, Lerner, SM, Brunzini, R, Evelson, P, Llesuy, S, 2009. Antioxidant status in the aqueous humour of patients with glaucoma associated with exfoliation syndrome. Eye, vol. 23, pp. 1691-7.

69. Holvoet, P, Harris, TB, Tracy, RP, 2003. Association of high coronary heart disease risk status with circulating oxidized LDL in the well functioning elderly: Findings from the health, aging, and body composition study. Arterioscler Thromb Vasc Biol, vol. 23, pp. 1444–8

70. Tanaga, K, Bujo, H, Inoue, M, 2002. Increased circulating malondialdehyde modified LDL levels in patients with coronary artery diseases and their association with peak sizes of LDL particles. Arterioscler Thromb Vasc Biol, vol. 22, pp. 662–6

71. Mehta, ML, Chen, J, Hermonat, RS, Romeo, F &Novelli, GT, 2006. Lectin-like, oxidized low-density lipoprotein receptor-1 (LOX-1): A critical player in the development of atherosclerosis and related disorders. Cardiovascular Research, vol. 69, pp. 36-45.

72. Gaut, JP, Hernecke, GW, 2007. Mechanism for oxidizing low-density lipoprotein. Trends Cardiovasc Med, vol. 16, pp. 103-12.

73 Kurnaz, O, Adyogan, HY, Isbir, CS, Tekeli, A, Isbir, T, 2009. Is LOX-1 K167N Polymorphism Protective for Coronary Artery Disease?. In vivo, vol. 23, pp. 969-74.

74. Lee, DY, Lee, MH, Jung, TS, Kwon, BW, Baek, NI, Rho, YD, 2010. Triterpenoid and Lignan from the Fruits of *Cornuskousa* inhibit the Activities of PRL-3 and LDL-Oxidation. J Korean Soc Appl Biol Chem, vol. 53, no. 1, pp. 97-100.

75. Maesen, L.J.G, van der and S. Sadikin, 1992. *Phaseolus vulgaris* L. Plant Resources of South-East Asia. Prosea, Bogor Indonesia. p. 60-3

76. Nainggolan, P., 2001. Sayuran Unggulan Di Lahan Kering Dataran Tinggi Sumatera Utara dan Arahan Teknologi. Balai Pengkajian Teknologi Pertanian Sumatera Utara, *Monograf*, Badan Penelitian dan Pengembangan Pertanian, Departemen Pertanian. Hal: 63-5

77. Cahyono, 2007. Kacang Buncis, Teknik Budidaya dan Analisis Usaha Tani. Penerbit Kanisius. Hal. 9-125

78. Rubatzky, V.E., 1997. Sayuran Dunia. Prinsip, Produksi, dan Gizi. Alih Bahasa Mas Yamaguchi, (1998) dari Judul Asli: Word Vegetables. Principles, Production, and Nutritive Values. ITB. Hal: 236-49

79. Tindall, H.D, 1983. Vegetables In The Tropics. The Macmillan Press, LTD London. p. 281-4

80. Mackay, S, Ball, MJ, 2002. Do beans and oat bran add to the effectiveness of a low fat diet ?. Eur J Clin Nutr, vol. 56, pp. 641-6

81. Verhaar, MC, Wever, RMF, Kastelein, JJP, Loon, DV, Milstien, S, Koomans HA, et al, 2009. Neuregulin-1 Is Associated With Disease Severity and Adverse Outcomes in Chronic Heart Failure. Circulation, vol. 120, pp. 335-8.

82. Brown, L, Rosner, B, Willett, WW, Sacks, FM, 2009. Cholesterol-lowering effects of dietary fiber : a meta-analysis. Am J Clin Nutr, vol. 78, pp. 30-42.

83. Nijveldt, RJ, Nood, EV, Hoorn, DEC, Boelens, PG, Norren, KV, Leeuwen PAM, 2001. Flavonoids: a review of probable mechanisms of action and potential applications. Am J Clin Nutr, vol. 74, pp. 418-25.

84. Hertog, MG, Feskens, EJ, Hollman, PC, Katan, MB, Kromhout, D, 2003. Dietary antioxidant flavonoids and risk of coronary heart disease: The Zutphen Elderly Study. Lancet, vol. 383, pp. 1007-11.

85. Halliwell, B, 2006. How to characterize an antioxidant: an update. BiochemSocSymp, vol. 69, pp. 73-101.

86. Joseph, JA, Shukitt-Hale, B, Denisova, NA, Prior, RL, Cao, GH, Martin, A, Taglialatela, G, Bickford, PC, 2009. Long-term dietary strawberry, spinach, or vitamin E supplementation retards the onset of age-related neuronal signal transduction and cognitive behavioural deficits. J. Neurosci. vol. 27, pp. 8047-55.

87. Joseph, JA, Shukitt-Hale, B, Denisova, NA, Bielinski, D, Martin, A, McEwen, JJ, Bickford, PC, 2007. Reversals of age-related declines in neuronal signal transduction; cognitive and behavioural deficits with blueberry, spinach or strawberry dietary supplementation. J. Neurosci, vol. 24, pp. 8114-21.

88. Cantutui-Castelvetri, I, Shukitt-Hale, B, Joseph, JA, 2010. Neurobehavioral aspects of antioxidants in aging. Int. J. Dev. Neurosci, vol. 26, pp. 367-81.

89. Cockle, SM, Kimbe, S, Hindmarch, I, 2008. The effects of *Gingko biloba*extract (LI 1370) supplementation on activities of daily living in free living older volunteers: a questionnaire survey. Hum. Psychopharm. Clin. vol. 21, pp. 227-35.

90. Bastianetto, S, Zheng, WH, Quirion, R, 2010. The *Gingko biloba*extract (Egb 761) protects and rescues hippocampal cells against nitric oxide-induced toxicity : Involvement of its flavonoids constituents and protein kinase C. J. Neurochem, vol. 79, pp. 2268-77.

91. Inanami, O, Watanabe, Y, Syuto, B, Nakano, M, Tsuji, M, Kuwabara, M, 2007. Oral administration of catechin protects against ischemia-reperfusion-induced neuronal death in the gerbil. Free Radical Res, vol. 38, pp. 359-65.

92. Schroeter, H, Spencer, J, Evans, CI, Williams, RJ, 2004. Flavonoids protect neurons from oxidized low-density-lipoprotein-induced apoptosis involving c-Jun N-terminal kinase (JNK), c-Jun and caspase-3. Biochem. J, vol. 362, pp, 547-57.

93. Roza, JM, Liu, ZX, Guthrie, N, 2007. Effects of citrus flavonoids and tocotrienols on serum cholesterol levels in hypercholesterolemic subjects. Altern Ther Health Med, vol. 13, no. 6, pp. 44-8.

94. Malinow, MR, Connor, WE, McLaughlin, P, Stafford, C, Lin, DS, Livingston, AL, 2004. Cholesterol and bile acid balance in *Macacafascicularis*. J Clin Invest, vol. 92, pp. 156-62.

95. Jeyakumar, SM, Vajreswari, A, Giridharan, NV, 2007. Impact of vitamin A on high-density lipoprotein-cholesterol and scavenger receptor class BI in the obese rat. Obesity, vol. 15, no. 2, pp. 322-9.

96. Mercodia, 2003. Test procedur for oxidied LDL ELISA, pp. 9.

97. Noviyanti, R, Syafruddin, D, Duffy, M, 2007. Manual of Methods. Isolasi DNA dari kertas saring dengan menggunakan Chelex-100. Jakarta, AIMRI, pp. 57.

98. Itabe, H, Obama, T, Kato, R, 2011. The Dynamics of Oxidized LDL during Atherogenesis. Journal of Lipids, vol, 2011, pp. 1-9.

99. Tsimikas, S, Aikawa, M, Miller, FJ, *et al*, 2007. Increased plasma oxidized phospholipids: apolipoprotein B-100 ratio with concomitant depletion of oxidized phospholipids from atherosclerotic lesions after dietary lipid-lowering : a potential biomarker of early atherosclerosis regression. Arteriosclerosis, Thrombosis, and Vascular Biology, vol. 27, no. 1, pp. 175-81.

100. Uno, M, Kitazato, T, Nishi, K, Itabe, H, Nagahiro, S, 2003. Raised plasma oxidized LDL in acute cerebral infarction, Journal of Neurology, Neurosurgery and Psychiatry, vol. 74, no. 3, pp. 312-6.

101. Yla–Herttuala, S, 2008. Is oxidized low-density lipoprotein present in vivo? CurrOpinLipidol. vol. 16, pp. 337–44.

102. Sentinelli, F, Filippi, E, Fallarino, M, Romeo, S, Fanelli, M, Buzzetti, R, et *al*, 2006. The 3'-UTR C>T polymorphism of the oxidized LDL-receptor 1 (OLR1) gene does not associate with coronary artery disease in Italian CAD patients or with the severity of coronary disease. Nutrition, Metabolism & Cardiovascular Diseases, vol. 16, pp. 345-52.

103. Silaste, ML, Rantala, M, Alfthan, G, Aro, A, WitztumJL, Kesaniemi, YA, et al, 2004. Changes in Dietary Fat Intake Alter Plasma Levels of Oxidized Low-Density Lipoprotein and Lipoprotein(a).. Arteriosclerosis Thrombosis Vascular Biology, vol, 24, pp. 498-503.

104. Omenn, GS, Goodman, GE, Thornquist, MD, Balmes, J, Cullen, MR, Glass, A, et al, 2006. Effects of a combination of beta carotene and vitamin A on lung cancer and cardiovascular disease. N Engl J Med, vol. 352, pp. 1150-55.

105. Hennekens, CH, Buring, JE, Manson, JE, Stampfer, M, Rosner, B, Cook, NR, et al, 2006. Lack of effect of long-term supplementation with beta carotene on the incidence of malignant neoplasms and cardiovascular disease. N Engl J Med, vol. 352, pp. 1145-49.

106. The Alpha-Tocopherol, Beta Carotene Cancer Prevention Study Group, 2004. The effect of vitamin E and beta carotene on the incidence of lung cancer and other cancers in male smokers. N Engl J Med, vol. 3580, pp. 1029-35.

107. Parthasarathy, S, Young, SG, Witztum, JL, Pittman, RC, Steinberg, D, 2006. Probucol inhibits oxidative modification of low density lipoprotein. J Clin Invest, vol. 94, pp. 641-4

108. Gruppo Italiano, 2009. Dietary supplementation with n-3 polyunsaturated fatty acids and vitamin E after myocardial infarction: results of the GISSI-Prevenzione trial. Lancet, vol. 402, pp. 447–55.

109. Lee, IM, Cook, NR, Gaziano, JM, Gordon, D, Ridker, PM, Manson JE, Hennekens, CH, Buring, JE, 2005. Vitamin E in the primary prevention of cardiovascular disease and cancer: the Women's Health Study: a randomized controlled trial. JAMA, vol. 294, pp. 56–65.

110. Steinberg, D, Witztum, JL, 2002. Is the Oxidative Modification Hypothesis Relevant to Human Atherosclerosis?. Circulation, vol. 105, pp. 2107-11.

111. Steinberg, D, Witztum, JL, 2010. History of Discovery. Oxidized Low-Density Lipoprotein and Atherosclerosis. Arteriosclerosis, Thrombosis, and Vascular Biology, vol. 30, pp. 2311-6.

112. Steinberg, D, 2009. The LDL modification hypothesis of atherogenesis: an update. Journal of Lipid Research, vol. 50, pp. S376-81.

113. Kris-Etherton, PM, Lichtenstein, AH, Howard, BV, Steinberg, D, Witztum, JL, 2004. Antioxidant Vitamin Supplements and Cardiovascular Disease.Circulation, vol. 110, pp. 637-41.

114. Tepel M, van der Giet M, Statz M, Jankowski J, Zidek W, 2003. The antioxidant acetylcysteine reduces cardiovascular events in patients with end-stage renal failure: a randomized, controlled trial. Circulation, vol. 107, pp. 992-5.

115. Milman U, Blum S, Shapira C, Aronson D, Miller-Lotan R, Anbinder Y, et al, 2008. Vitamin E supplementation reduces cardiovascular events in a subgroup of middle-aged individuals with both type 2 diabetes mellitus and the haptoglobin 2–2 genotype: a prospective double-blinded clinical trial. Arteriosclerosis, Thrombosis, and Vascular Biology, vol. 28, pp. 341-7.

116. Fang, R, Zhang, N, Wang, C, Zhao, X, Liu, L, Wang, Y, et al, 2011. Relations between plasma Ox-LDL and carotid plaque among Chinese Han ethnic group. Neurological Research, vol, 33, no.5, pp. 460-6.

117. Itabe, H, Ueda, M, 2007. Measurement of Plasma Oxidized Low-Density Lipoprotein and its Clinical Implications. Journal of Atherosclerosis and Thrombosis, vol, 14, no. 1, pp. 1-11.

118. Nishi, K, Itabe, H, Uno M, 2002. Oxidized LDL in carotid plaques and plasma associates with plaque instability. Arterioscler Thromb Vasc Biol, vol. 22, pp. 1649–54

119. Naruko, T, Ueda, M, Ehara, S, et al, 2006. Persistent high levels of plasme oxidized low-density lipoprotein after acute myocardial infarction predict stent restenosis. Arteriosclerosis, Thrombosis, and Vascular Biology, vol. 26, no. 4, pp. 877-83.

120. Garrido-Sanchez, L, García-Almeida, JM, García-Serrano, S, Cardona, I, García-Arnes, J, Soriguer, F, et al., 2008. Improved Carbohydrate Metabolism After Bariatric Surgery Raises Antioxidized LDL Antibody Levels in Morbidly Obese Patients. Diabetes Care, vol. 31, pp. 2258–64.

121. Regnstro, J, Nilsson, J, Tornvall, P, Landou C, Hamsten A, 2003. Susceptibility to low-density lipoprotein oxidation and coronary atherosclerosis in man. Lancet, vol. 428, pp. 1183–6.

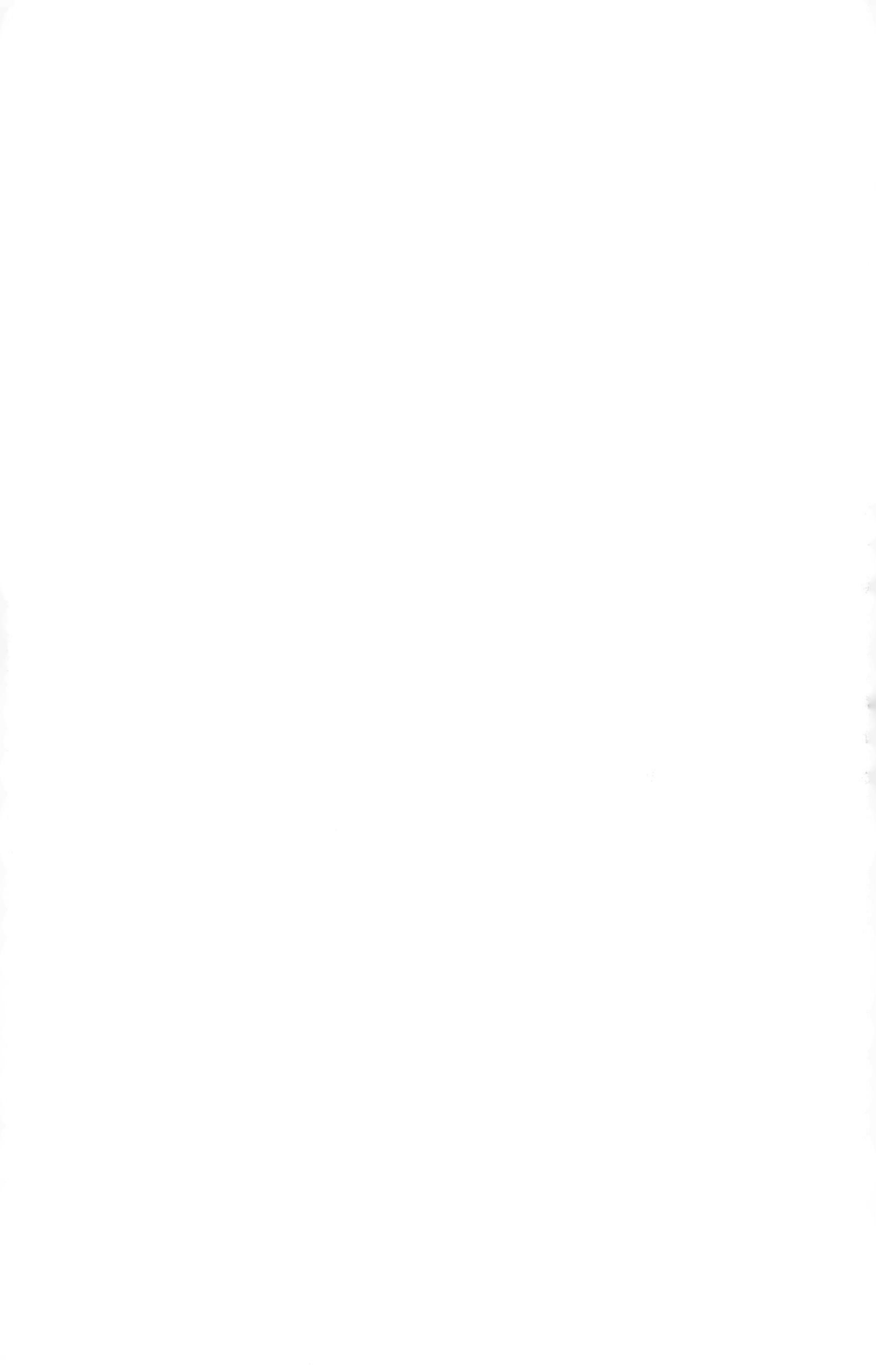

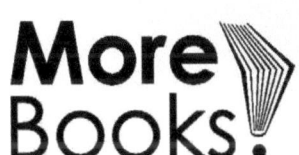
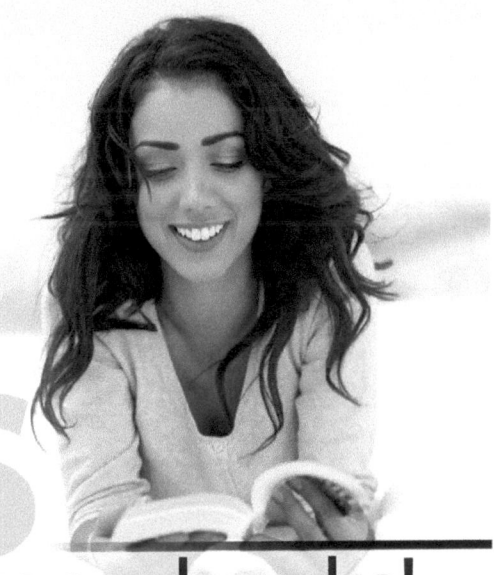
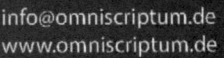
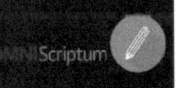

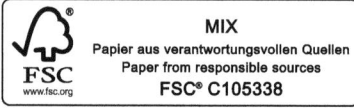
Printed by Books on Demand GmbH, Norderstedt / Germany